Contents

Introduction

Before the medical community had better understanding of the mechanisms that cause disease, doctors believed certain ailments could originate from imbalances in the stomach. This was called hypochondriasis. (In Ancient Greek, hypochondrium refers to the upper part of the abdomen, the region between the breastbone and the navel.) This concept was rejected as science evolved and, for example, we could look under a microscope and see bacteria, parasites, and viruses. The meaning of the term changed, and for many years, doctors used the word "hypochondriac" to describe a person who has a persistent, often inexplicable fear of having a serious medical illness.

But what if this ancient concept of illnesses originating in the gut actually holds some truth? Could some of the chronic diseases our society faces today actually be associated with a dysfunctional gastrointestinal system.

The expression "leaky gut" is getting a lot of attention in medical blogs and social media lately, but don't be surprised if your doctor does not recognize this term. Leaky gut, also called increased intestinal permeability, is somewhat new and most of the research occurs in basic sciences. However, there is growing interest to develop medications that may be used in patients to combat the effects of this problem.

Inside our bellies, we have an extensive intestinal lining covering more than 4,000 square feet of surface area. When working properly, it forms a tight barrier that controls what gets absorbed into the bloodstream. An unhealthy gut lining may have large cracks or holes, allowing partially digested food, toxins, and bugs to penetrate the tissues beneath it. This may trigger inflammation and changes in the gut flora (normal bacteria) that could lead to problems within the digestive tract and beyond. The research world is booming today with studies showing that modifications in the intestinal bacteria and inflammation may play a role in the development of several common chronic diseases.

We all have some degree of leaky gut, as this barrier is not completely impenetrable (and isn't supposed to be!).

Some of us may have a genetic predisposition and may be more sensitive to changes in the digestive system, but our DNA is not the only one to blame. Modern life may actually be the main driver of gut inflammation. There is emerging evidence that the standard American diet, which is low in fiber and high in sugar and saturated fats, may initiate this process. Heavy alcohol use and stress also seem to disrupt this balance.

We already know that increased intestinal permeability plays a role in certain gastrointestinal conditions such as celiac disease, Crohn's disease, and irritable bowel syndrome. The biggest question is whether or not a leaky gut may cause problems elsewhere in the body. Some studies show that leaky gut may be associated with other autoimmune diseases (lupus, type 1 diabetes, multiple sclerosis), chronic fatigue syndrome, fibromyalgia, arthritis, allergies, asthma, acne, obesity, and even mental illness. However, we do not yet have clinical studies in humans showing such a cause and effect.

Leaky Gut

The human digestive tract is where food is broken down and nutrients are absorbed.

The digestive system also plays an important role in protecting your body from harmful substances. The walls of the intestines act as barriers, controlling what enters the bloodstream to be transported to your organs.

Small gaps in the intestinal wall called tight junctions allow water and nutrients to pass through, while blocking the passage of harmful substances. Intestinal permeability refers to how easily substances pass through the intestinal wall.

When the tight junctions of intestinal walls become loose, the gut becomes more permeable, which may allow bacteria and toxins to pass from the gut into the bloodstream. This phenomenon is commonly referred to as "leaky gut."

When the gut is "leaky" and bacteria and toxins enter the bloodstream, it can cause widespread inflammation and possibly trigger a reaction from the immune system.

Supposed symptoms of leaky gut syndrome include bloating, food sensitivities, fatigue, digestive issues and skin problems.

However, leaky gut is not a recognized medical diagnosis. In fact, some medical professionals deny that it even exists. Proponents claim that it's the underlying cause of all sorts of conditions, including chronic fatigue syndrome, migraines, multiple sclerosis, fibromyalgia, food sensitivities, thyroid abnormalities, mood swings, skin conditions and autism.

The problem is that very few scientific studies mention leaky gut syndrome.

Nevertheless, medical professionals do agree that increased intestinal permeability, or intestinal hyperpermeability, exists in certain chronic diseases.

Leaky gut, or intestinal hyperpermeability, is a phenomenon that occurs when the tight junctions of the intestinal wall become loose, allowing harmful substances to enter the bloodstream.

Symptoms of Leaky Gut

Leaky gut shares many of its symptoms with other health conditions. This can make the condition difficult for doctors to identify.

Leaky gut may cause or contribute to the following symptoms:

- chronic diarrhea, constipation, or bloating
- nutritional deficiencies
- fatigue
- headaches
- confusion
- difficulty concentrating
- skin problems, such as acne, rashes, or eczema
- joint pain
- widespread inflammation

Causes Leaky Gut

Leaky gut syndrome remains a bit of a medical mystery, and medical professionals are still trying to determine exactly what causes it.A protein called zonulin is the only known regulator of intestinal permeability.When it's activated in genetically susceptible people, it can lead to leaky gut. Two factors that trigger the release of zonulin are bacteria in the intestines and gluten, which is a protein found in wheat and other grains.

While there are still a lot of unanswered questions about what exactly causes the condition in the first place, poor diet choices, chronic stress, an overabundance of toxins in the system, and bacterial imbalances can all wreak havoc on your health. Ongoing research is emerging that connects common health concerns and chronic issues to leaky gut syndrome, so one thing is clear: This isn't a problem that can be flushed down the toilet. many things can trigger leaky gut syndrome. These can include inflammatory bowel disease, nonsteroidal anti-inflammatory drugs (NSAID), overgrown bacteria in the small intestine, fungal dysbiosis (which is similar to a candida yeast overgrowth), celiac disease, parasitic infections, alcohol, food allergies, aging, excessive exercise, and nutritional deficiencies.

Gluten is one of the biggest contributors to a leaky gut, due to its release of a chemical called zonulin. This protein regulates the bonds, called tight junctions, at the intersections of the gut lining. Excess zonulin can signal the lining cells to open, weakening the bond and causing symptoms of leaky gut.zonulin is linked to impaired gut barrier function in relation to several diseases, including autoimmune and neurodegenerative conditions.

There are likely multiple contributing factors to leaky gut syndrome.

Below are a few factors that are believed to play a role:

1. Excessive sugar intake: An unhealthy diet high in sugar, particularly fructose, harms the barrier function of the intestinal wall.

2. Non-steroidal anti-inflammatory drugs (NSAIDs): The long-term use of NSAIDs like ibuprofen can

increase intestinal permeability and contribute to leaky gut.

3. Excessive alcohol intake: Excessive alcohol intake may increase intestinal permeability.

4. Nutrient deficiencies: Deficiencies in vitamin A, vitamin D and zinc have each been implicated in increased intestinal permeability.

5. Inflammation: Chronic inflammation throughout the body can contribute to leaky gut syndrome.

6. Stress: Chronic stress is a contributing factor to multiple gastrointestinal disorders, including leaky gut.

7. Poor gut health: There are millions of bacteria in the gut, some beneficial and some harmful. When the balance between the two is disrupted, it can affect the barrier function of the intestinal wall.

8. Yeast overgrowth: Yeast is naturally present in the gut, but an overgrowth of yeast may contribute to leaky gut,

Medical professionals are still trying to determine what causes leaky gut syndrome. An unhealthy diet, long-term

NSAID use, stress and chronic inflammation are some factors that are believed to contribute to it.

Diseases Associated With Leaky Gut

The claim that leaky gut is the root of modern health problems has yet to be proven by science. However, many studies have connected increased intestinal permeability with multiple chronic diseases.

Celiac Disease

Celiac disease is an autoimmune disease characterized by a severe sensitivity to gluten. Intestinal permeability is higher in patients with celiac disease.

In fact, one study found that ingesting gluten significantly increases intestinal permeability in celiac patients immediately after consumption.

Diabetes

There is some evidence that increased intestinal permeability plays a role in the development of type 1 diabetes. Type 1 diabetes is caused by an autoimmune destruction of insulin-producing beta cells in the pancreas .

It has been suggested that the immune reaction responsible for beta cell destruction may be triggered by foreign substances "leaking" through the gut.

42% of individuals with type 1 diabetes had significantly elevated zonulin levels. Zonulin is a known moderator of intestinal permeability.

In animals, rats that developed diabetes were found to have abnormal intestinal permeability prior to developing diabetes.

Crohn's Disease

Increased intestinal permeability plays a significant role in Crohn's disease. Crohn's is a chronic digestive disorder characterized by persistent inflammation of the intestinal tract.

Several studies have observed an increase in intestinal permeability in patients with Crohn's disease.

A few studies also found increased intestinal permeability in relatives of Crohn's patients, who are at an increased risk of developing the disease.

This suggests that increased permeability may be connected to the genetic component of Crohn's disease.

Irritable Bowel Syndrome
People with irritable bowel syndrome (IBS) are likely to have increased intestinal permeability.

IBS is a digestive disorder characterized by both diarrhea and constipation.One study found that increased intestinal permeability is particularly prevalent in those with diarrhea-predominant IBS.

Food Allergies
A few studies have shown that individuals with food allergies often have impaired intestinal barrier function.

A leaky gut may allow food proteins to cross the intestinal barrier, stimulating an immune response. An immune response to a food protein, which is known as an antigen, is the definition of a food allergy.

Multiple studies have demonstrated that increased intestinal permeability is indeed present in people with certain chronic diseases.

Leaky Gut a Cause or Symptom of Disease
Proponents of leaky gut syndrome claim it's the underlying cause of most modern health problems.

Indeed, plenty of studies have shown that increased intestinal permeability is present in several chronic diseases, specifically autoimmune disorders.

However, it is difficult to prove that leaky gut is the cause of disease.

Skeptics argue that increased intestinal permeability is a symptom of chronic disease, rather than an underlying cause (34).

Interestingly, animal studies on celiac disease, type 1 diabetes and IBS have identified increased intestinal permeability prior to the onset of disease.

This evidence supports the theory that leaky gut is involved in the development of disease.

On the other hand, a study found that intestinal permeability in people with celiac disease returned to normal in 87% of people who followed a gluten-free diet for over a year.A gluten-free diet is the standard treatment for celiac disease.

This suggests that the abnormal intestinal permeability may be a response to gluten ingestion, rather than the cause of celiac disease.

Overall, there is not yet sufficient evidence to prove that leaky gut is the underlying cause of chronic diseases.increased intestinal permeability is present in several chronic conditions. However, there is no conclusive evidence that leaky gut is the underlying cause of them.

Some Claims About Leaky Gut Syndrome

There is enough evidence to demonstrate that leaky gut syndrome does exist. However, some of the claims being made are not backed by science.

Proponents of leaky gut have claimed that it's connected to a wide variety of ailments, including autism, anxiety, depression, eczema and cancer. Most of these claims have yet to be proven by scientific studies.

A proportion of autistic children have increased intestinal permeability, but other studies have found that intestinal permeability was normal.

Currently, there are no studies that show leaky gut presence prior to the onset of autism, which means there is no evidence that it is a causative factor.

There is some evidence that bacteria crossing the intestinal wall may play a role in anxiety and depression, but more research is needed to prove this possible connection.

Furthermore, some of the proposed treatments for leaky gut syndrome have weak scientific support.

Many supplements and remedies being sold by websites have not yet been proven to be effective.

Treatment and improving gut health
Exercising regularly can help improve digestion.

Since many doctors do not consider leaky gut to be a legitimate medical condition, there is no standard treatment.

However, certain dietary and lifestyle changes may help people to improve their gut health. This, in turn, may alleviate leaky gut symptoms.

The following dietary tips may help to improve gut health:

- eating more probiotics to boost beneficial gut bacteria
- eating foods rich in prebiotic fiber, such as vegetables and whole grains

- eating less meat, dairy, and eggs

- avoiding added sugar and artificial sweeteners

The following lifestyle changes can improve digestion and support a healthy gut:

- exercising regularly

- getting enough sleep every night

- reducing stress

- avoiding unnecessary use of antibiotics

- quitting smoking

Leaky Gut Diet

Gut health refers to the balance of microorganisms that live in the digestive tract. There's a delicate balance of essential microbes in the gut, and this balance is critical!

The spheres of modern life such as little sleep, eating processed high sugar foods, and even anxiety can upset your 'gut feeling' or, as the experts call it, the gut microbiome.

The optimum balance of these microorganisms is what ensures desirable physical health, mental health, and immunity.

A basic overview of the digestive process
Digestion works by passing food through the GI (gastrointestinal) tract. It starts right when you chew the first morsel of food and ends in the small intestine.

As the food passes through the GI tract, blending takes place- food passing through with essential digestive juices, causing huge molecules of food to disintegrate into smaller bits or molecules.

The body then imbibes these smaller molecules through the thin walls of the small intestine into the bloodstream.

Your blood performs the function of delivering nutrition to the rest of the body, leaving the waste products of the digestion process which passes through the large intestine and then out of your body as a solid matter (stool).

Importance of gut health

When your gut health isn't right, bloating, diarrhea, stomach pain for no reason, and many other conditions can occur, seemingly out of nowhere. When a person's microbiome is thrown out of function, he or she can suffer from physical problems.

Inflammatory bowel diseases (IBD's) like Crohn's disease can affect any area of the gastrointestinal tract, from the mouth to the anus, either in continuity or as isolated areas. If these diseases permeate the intestines, it can impair GI function.

Even anxiety and depression put GI impairment into effect. The functionality of a person's gut is directly proportional to the diversity of the gut microbiome.

Gut microbes

Gut microbes are a collection of bacteria, viruses, fungi and other microorganisms, which contrary to popular belief based on stigmas, are actually good for keeping your gut happy. Common examples include lactobacillus and bifidobacterium, which have a pronounced probiotic function.

Out of all these microscopic living things, bacteria are the most vastly studied. There are more bacteria in your body than cells!

Hence, foods promoting the growth of these beneficial microbiota are the key for a healthy gut. The more diverse your gut microbiome is, the healthier your body will feel. Diversity comes from eating foods which contain a vast variety of bacteria with many of them, specifically healing the body by performing various functions.

Foods to avoid when you have a leaky gut.
While gluten is often called out as the main cause of a leaky gut, experts also point to other pro-inflammatory foods as possible culprits. Eliminate the following foods from your diet if you suspect you have a leaky gut:

Gluten

Because gluten is linked to the release of zonulin, it tops most doctors' lists of leaky-gut-causing foods.Common sources of gluten include pastas, noodles, breads, pastries, cereal, granola, and beer (or any malt beverage).

Sugar

This includes not just refined sugars like high-fructose corn syrup but also seemingly "healthy" sweeteners like monk fruit and coconut sugar. Even alcoholic beverages break down as sugar. These wreak havoc in your gut, and research shows sugar can feed bad gut bacteria.

Dairy products

This includes milk, yogurt, ice cream, and cheese.Specifically, there are two proteins in dairy that many people struggle to digest—casein and whey. Additionally, many people don't have enough lactase to properly break down the lactose in milk, which can lead to gastrointestinal distress and potential gut damage.

Soy products

Soy and its derivatives can be found in everything from tofu to edamame, protein bars, and even some nutritional supplements. Soy may trigger gut flora imbalances, and is commonly genetically modified. Many experts recommend avoiding genetically modified foods as much as possible if you have a leaky gut.

Corn

More than 90% of the corn grown in the United States is reportedly genetically modified. It's also a food to which many people (especially those with leaky guts) can develop a sensitivity. The effects of a corn sensitivity are similar to those of a gluten sensitivity. Like gluten and soy, corn is present in many packaged foods, so it's important to read labels carefully.

Lectins and phytates

These compounds are found in all gluten-containing grains. Lectins are also found in beans, corn, and nightshade vegetables like tomatoes, eggplant, peppers, and potatoes. Lectins may bind to the cells lining your intestines, disrupting the tight junctions between the intestinal cells, contributing to leaky gut, while phytates can interfere with the absorption of important minerals. It can be useful to scale back on these foods and see if symptoms improve.

Foods to eat when you have a leaky gut.
Now that you know what not to eat, you might be thinking, "What's left?" "Focus on clean ingredients with easy-to-digest foods that are low in fructose and sugar and devoid of any substances, including sugar alcohols and pesticides, that are hard on the gut," Pedre told mbg. Want more specifics? Below are the basic components of a gut-friendly diet:

Healthy fats
Go for quality fat sources like nuts, seeds, avocado, olive oil, and coconut oil. Skip ultra-refined vegetable oils like corn and soybean, which can promote inflammation.

High-fiber, low-glycemic carbs
High-fiber foods can also work as prebiotics. They help feed the microorganisms and create their source of energy called short-chain fatty acids (SCFAs).These include nonstarchy vegetables. Think leafy greens and

cruciferous vegetables such as arugula, broccoli, Brussels sprouts, cabbage, cauliflower, and collard greens. These are a great source of prebiotic fiber, which can help feed the healthy probiotic bacteria in your gut, which are essential to gut health. You may also want to focus on foods high in resistant starch (e.g. beans, peas, lentils). This is the type of starch that "escapes" digestion and goes directly to the large intestine.

1. Broccoli

Broccoli is an excellent anti-inflammatory.Not only is it good for you, but it has loads of vitamins, flavonoids, and carotenoids, which is great for an anti-inflammatory diet. You should always steam your broccoli before you eat it, as research has shown added health benefits in doing so.

2. Avocado

Avocado is an anti-inflammatory, and it comes by it naturally. It is one of the best non-animal fats for your digestive system and will have you well on your way to digestive health by keeping your body full of healthy and lean fat.

3. Salmon

Salmon is rich in Omega-3 fatty acids, which helps cushion the joints, fight inflammation and keeps your brain healthy. Salmon is also loaded with lean fats and Omega-6 and Omega-9, all of which help support a healthy overall body.

If you suffer from joint or arthritis pain, eating salmon can help ease it due to the high concentration of oil.

Salmon also contains high doses of protein and B vitamins and may be useful in helping you manage obesity and keep you staying slim.

4. Walnuts

Whether you choose walnut salads, walnut recipes or just snacking on a handful whenever you get the urge, these nuts are packed with phytonutrients that no other nuts have.

Walnuts are also high in Omega-3 fatty acids, which, like salmon, can help with inflammation and cushion joints that are feeling sore from arthritis.

They can also provide an excellent source of protein and healthy fats to your diet.

5. Blueberries

Blueberries are rich in antioxidants and anti-inflammatory properties, which can help heal your leaky gut. They also contain an amazing antioxidant, quercetin, which can help protect the body from a host of diseases.

They are also rich in Vitamins A, C, and K and contain several grams of fiber. Fiber-rich foods are an important part of healing your leaky gut, and blueberries can play an excellent role.

Slow carbs
Think starchy vegetables such as sweet potatoes and butternut squash; fiber-rich, low-sugar fruits like apples and berries; and minimally processed, fiber-rich grains like rolled oats instead of breads and refined grains.

These are less likely to contain anti-nutrients like lectins and phytates that can aggravate the gut.

Hypoallergenic proteins
These include pea, rice, hemp, chia. A leaky gut makes people more prone to food allergies and sensitivities, meaning it's a good general practice to go hypoallergenic when possible.

Clean and lean proteins
Compared to their conventional counterparts, free-range poultry, wild-caught fish, and grass-fed meats contain healthier concentrations of omega-3 fats, which are anti-inflammatory.

Bone broth (or collagen)
The gelatin in bone broth protects and heals the mucosal lining of the digestive tract and helps aid in the digestion of nutrients. Some research suggests collagen peptides may have a similar benefit. Bone broth is also a rich source of glutamine, an amino acid that's a preferred source of energy for the cells of the small bowel and other immune cells and that has been shown to reduce intestinal permeability. Want a vegan alternative?

Galangal broth, a traditional Chinese medicine remedy, may also help heal a leaky gut.

Fermented foods

Foods like kimchi, unpasteurized sauerkraut, and lacto-fermented pickles are all rich sources of probiotics that help keep your immune system strong, fend off pathogens, and protect the gut lining.These are tangy or sour foods whose composition changed by adding lactic acid bacteria. They are among the best foods for a diet for leaky gut because they are rich in probiotics.

Probiotics refer to foods that introduce live microorganisms into the intestines. Their purpose is to improve the diversity or number of good bacteria in the gut.

Some examples of fermented foods are:

- Kimchi, a popular Korean side dish
- Sauerkraut, which is fermented cabbage
- Kombucha or fermented tea

Kefir or fermented dairy (sometimes kefir may be from fruit or vegetable)

Miso, which is from fermented soybeans

Note: While probiotic-rich foods are healthy, they may have only one or a few strains of bacteria. Since diversity is essential for an excellent microbiome, supplement your leaky gut diet with BIOHM Probiotics.

Important note: If you suspect that your leaky gut is caused by IBS, or if your symptoms don't improve when eating the foods suggested above, you may need a stricter approach called a low-FODMAP diet to heal properly.

Lifestyle habits for leaky gut.
Changing your diet is the first step, but to further support your gut, consider the following:

Add a probiotic supplement: Good gut bacteria, which are crucial in preventing leaky gut, can become depleted or disrupted by a number of things (poor diet, antibiotics, steroids, antacids, etc.), and fermented foods may not deliver the amount you need. So, taking a highly concentrated probiotic (25 to 100 billion units) daily may help you support a healthy balance of bacteria in your gut.

Reduce your use of NSAIDs: This class of anti-inflammatory pain relievers is notoriously harsh on the stomach, and research suggests that taking them too frequently may increase the risk of intestinal permeability. So, for minor aches and pains that don't require serious intervention, consider popping a gentle, natural anti-inflammatory like turmeric.

Find healthy ways to de-stress: Our anxious thoughts can have a direct impact on things like digestion and overall gut health. So, it's no surprise that chronic stress has been associated with increased intestinal permeability, or leaky gut. Try to do something that helps you chill on a regular basis. Yoga, meditation, progressive muscle relaxation, deep breathing, and body scanning are all great options.

Foods For Improved Gut Health

Knowing the correct supplements is a must, especially when our food intake decides which kind of microorganisms thrive in our body. Here are 10 foods which can prove to be a boon for your gut health.

Miso

Miso means fermented beans in Japanese. It is made from fermented soybeans and contains billions of beneficial bacteria. In Japan, many people still begin their day with a hearty bowl of miso soup to stimulate digestion and energize the body.

Miso is quite rich in essential minerals and a great source of vitamins (B, E, and K) and folic acid. It also adds the fifth element of taste (umami) to dishes like soups, broths, stews, and marinades.

Oryzae is the most important probiotic strain found in miso. Research shows that the probiotics in this condiment may help reduce symptoms linked to digestive problems, including inflammatory bowel disease (IBD).

Plant-based metabolic enzymes and probiotics, which are abundantly found in miso, can survive the journey through your intestines. They have a higher heat resistance than animal-based probiotics like the ones in most yogurts.

There's no wonder that this Japanese superfood is being highly recommended for gut health.

Kimchi
Kimchi is a traditional Korean dish made by lacto-fermentation, which is also responsible for other fermented delicacies like sauerkraut (more on that later!). In the primary stage, cabbage is soaked in a salty brine that eliminates harmful bacteria.

In the next step, the surviving Lactobacillus bacteria (good bacteria) mentioned earlier as well, convert sugars into lactic acid, which preserves the vegetables and imparts flavor.

Gut-friendly bacteria can allow the production of chemicals called short-chain fatty acids, which improves the immune system by keeping it balanced.

Gut bacteria need a stable and friendly environment in which to thrive. The ideal pH in the human colon is between 6.7 and 6.9. To sustain good bacteria and to prevent harmful bacteria from flourishing, the colon needs to be slightly acidic.

One of the easiest ways to maintain a desirable pH balance is to eat fruits high in fiber. The following fruits are highly effective:

Bananas

Bananas are highly rich in soluble fiber. They also contain a prebiotic compound that passes through the upper part of the gastrointestinal tract and remains undigested. Only when they pass through the small intestine, they reach the colon where they are fermented by the gut microflora.

Bananas maintain harmony among microbes in your intestinal ecosystem.

Raspberries

Raspberries are full of soluble fiber. The high fiber and water content in raspberries help prevent constipation and maintain a healthy digestive tract.

Pears

When it comes to our GI health, pears are fiber-dense fruits, and their skin is particularly beneficial. They contain at least three to four times as many phenolic phytonutrients as the flesh. These phytonutrients include antioxidants, anti-inflammatory flavonoids, and anti-carcinogenic phytonutrients, like cinnamic acids.

Apple

Apart from the other health benefits that apples are known for, intake of apples significantly alters amounts of two bacteria (clostridiales and bacteroides) in the large intestine. The balance of these bacteria has a significant impact on your metabolism.

Kiwi

The fiber in kiwi binds and removes toxins from the colon, which is beneficial in preventing colon cancer.They are also dense with nutrients like proteins with almost negligible fat value.

Blueberries

Keeping aside all the mouth-watering pies this fruit yields by its mere presence, blueberries are a major source of the bifidobacteria, which improves gut health. It has an important role in the process of digestion and is an abundant supply of the prebiotics contributing to the healthy bacteria in the gut and colon. No doubt, this one proves to be an essential part of the healthy gut food chart.

Sauerkraut

Sauerkraut (sour cabbage) is a German delicacy made from finely cut raw cabbage that has been fermented by various lactic acid bacteria. It has an enduring shelf life and a distinctive sour flavor.

Regularly eating sauerkraut can help reduce symptoms of the annoying Irritable Bowel Syndrome (IBS). It has also been noticed to cause a spike in good bacteria.

Sauerkraut contains dietary fiber which aids digestion, optimizes blood sugar, and may even help lower cholesterol. It contains far more lactobacillus than yogurt, making it a better probiotic.

A serving or two of sauerkraut every few days may help treat ulcerative colitis and irritable bowel syndrome.

Tempeh
Tempeh is a traditional Indonesian fermented soy product that's a popular vegetarian meat replacement. Tempeh is high in protein, prebiotics, and a wide array of vitamins and minerals.

Some studies have linked prebiotic intake with increased stool frequency, reduced inflammation, and improved memory.There's also evidence to show that drinking tempeh causes beneficial changes in the gut microbiota, the bacteria that reside in your digestive system.

Kefir
Kefir is a healthy drink which originated in Eastern Europe and Russia. Traditionally, kefir is fermented at ambient temperatures overnight. Active fermentation of

lactose yields a sour, carbonated, slightly alcoholic beverage. It is an effective antibiotic and helps with a lot of digestive system disorders.

It has a consistency and taste similar to drinkable yogurt, similar to lassi in India. However, like sauerkraut, it proves to be a more powerful probiotic than yogurt. Kefir can contain up to 30 strains of beneficial bacteria and yeasts. Some of the major strains include the lactobacillales or lactic acid bacteria, which is a good bacteria for our gut.

Broccoli

Broccoli, a nutritious cruciferous vegetable, is a member of the cabbage family. The cruciferous family of vegetables also includes cauliflower, brussel sprouts, arugula, bok choy, cabbage, kale, collard greens, cress, radishes, turnips, and kohlrabi.

Eating broccoli can help reduce inflammation in the colon and may decrease the incidence of colon cancer, among other cancers. It is also a source of folic acid which increases the appetite. With its relatively mild flavor, versatility, and affordability, broccoli provides an accessible and delicious way to give your body a brassica boost.

Dandelion Greens
Dandelion greens were historically used to purify the blood, address digestion-related problems, and prevent piles and gallstones. Dandelion greens are rich in inulin and pectin, which are soluble fibers that may help your body feel full longer and assist with weight control.

They might taste slightly bitter, so consider sautéing them with onions, drinking them with tea, or adding them to soups and salads.

Seaweed Jicama
Seaweed is high in fiber [25–75%]. This is higher than the fiber content of most fruits and vegetables.

Apart from its contribution to gut health, seaweed contains iodine and tyrosine, which support the thyroid function in our body and repair the damaged cells due to its unique calibre to absorb concentrated amounts of idonine from the ocean.

Fermentation of flaxseed fibers in the gut changes the microbiota to improve metabolic health and protect against diet-induced obesity.

Our data suggest that flaxseed fiber supplementation affects host metabolism by increasing energy expenditure and reducing obesity as well as by improving glucose tolerance. Future research should be directed to understand the relative contribution of the different microbes and delineate underlying mechanisms for how flaxseed fibers affect host metabolism.

A one-day leaky gut diet meal plan.

To get started on a leaky gut diet try this sample menu, but feel free to mix and match or swap in foods from the list above:

Breakfast: A couple of scrambled eggs with a side of sautéed kale. (pro tip: Cooked veggies are gentler on the gut and may be a better choice than raw when starting a leaky gut diet). Want something sweet? Go for a bowl of oatmeal with almond milk, berries, and walnuts.

Lunch: A salad with lentils and lean protein will provide sustained energy and a good dose of prebiotic fiber. Add some kimchi or sauerkraut for a probiotic boost. Salads not your thing? Scoop some tuna or chicken salad (made with an avocado-oil-based mayo) into romaine lettuce and eat it like a taco!

Snack: Carrot slices with hummus, apple slices with almond butter, or crunchy roasted chickpeas: The possibilities are endless, but leaky-gut-friendly snacks should include some gut-friendly fiber along with a bit of fat and protein to promote stable blood sugar.

Dinner: Think of this simple formula: Quality protein source + nonstarchy veggie + starchy veggie (optional) + healthy fat. Pan-seared salmon and roasted sweet potato and Brussels sprouts cooked in olive oil would fit the bill. Another option, Zucchini noodles with pesto, sun-dried tomatoes, and grilled chicken.

How to Improve Your Gut Health

Leaky gut syndrome is not an official medical diagnosis and there is not yet a recommended course of treatment.

Nevertheless, there are steps you can take to improve your gut health. One of the keys to a healthier gut is increasing the number of beneficial bacteria in it.

Limit your refined carb intake: Harmful bacteria thrive on sugar, and excessive sugar intake can harm gut barrier function.

Take a probiotic supplement: Probiotics are beneficial bacteria that can improve your gut health. Probiotic supplements have been shown to be beneficial for gastrointestinal diseases.

Eat fermented foods: Fermented foods, such as plain yogurt, kimchi, sauerkraut, kefir and kombucha, contain probiotics that can improve gut health.

Eat plenty of high-fiber foods: Soluble fiber, which is found in fruits, vegetables and legumes, feed the beneficial bacteria in your gut.

Limit the use of NSAIDs: The long-term use of NSAIDs like ibuprofen contributes to leaky gut syndrome

Conclusion

Leaky gut syndrome is a condition in which the cellular junctions of the intestinal wall become damaged, allowing undigested food and bacteria to "leak" into the bloodstream. Leaky gut has been implicated in many autoimmune disorders like IBS and celiac disease. However, it is not yet a widely recognized medical condition and more research is needed to understand the cause and proper treatment methods.

Although leaky gut syndrome is not well understood, there is evidence that a "leaky gut diet" can help alleviate symptoms. Avoiding gluten, dairy, sugar, and other common irritants, while focusing on healthy fats, fermented foods, probiotic supplements, and lifestyle factors can help heal the gut.

There is sufficient evidence to demonstrate that leaky gut syndrome exists. However, science has not yet proven that conditions like autism or cancer are related to leaky gut syndrome.